WHO COULD HAVE
IMAGINED!

WHO COULD HAVE IMAGINED!

MY STEVENS-JOHNSON SYNDROME EXPERIENCE

MICHELE MOORE

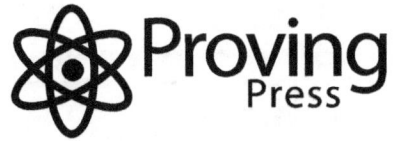

Book Design & Production
Columbus Publishing Lab
www.ColumbusPublishingLab.com

Copyright © 2018 by Michele Moore
LCCN 2018930941

All rights reserved. This book, or parts thereof, may not be reproduced in any form without permission.

Print ISBN: 978-1-63337-189-7
E-book ISBN: 978-1-63337-190-3

Printed in the United States of America
1 3 5 7 9 10 8 6 4 2

CONTENTS

Preface 1

Part One: Stevens-Johnson Syndrome 3

Part Two: Feeling Ill 5

Part Three: Too Weak 8

Part Four: What a Ride 12

Part Five: The Poison 15

Part Six: Have Faith 19

Part Seven: The Discovery 24

Part Eight: Medication List 28

Part Nine: Are You Sure 32

Part Ten: Visitors 35

Part Eleven: The Turn Around 42

Part Twelve: Home 46

Part Thirteen: The Conclusion 55

Acknowledgments 56

Photos 58

PREFACE

I always wanted to write a book, but I thought it would be on my life-growing experiences. But God! He changed things around and decided to have me tell the world about Stevens-Johnson Syndrome, acknowledge my own spiritual walk and the encounters and events that followed. Through others it was suggested that I write about my experiences for awareness. Awareness about your body and medications, awareness that throughout your experiences in life you might be approached several times by those who offer well-intentioned advice, but ultimately it might not be fully what God is trying to teach you at that moment. This is ok; just listen to them and ask God yourself what message He is trying to give you, and ask for that message to be clear with understanding so you can handle the instructions. He will do it, I promise! He will provide awareness of the procedure that could save your life or someone else's life. But most of all, the awareness that God is still the God who sits high and looks low. He still gives us signs when there is a need, and if your heart and eyes are focused on Him, you will recognize them without any questions in your mind. Now go, act on them!

✝

Part One
STEVENS-JOHNSON SYNDROME

What is Stevens-Johnson Syndrome?

Stevens-Johnson Syndrome (SJS) is an immune complex mediated hypersensitivity complex that typically involves the skin and mucous membranes. While minor presentations may occur, significant involvement of oral, nasal, ocular, vaginal, urethral, gastrointestinal, and lower respiratory involvement may progress to necrosis. Stevens-Johnson Syndrome is a serious systemic disorder with potential for severe morbidity and even death.

Stevens-Johnson Syndrome is a form of toxic epidermal necrolysis—a life-threatening skin condition—in which cell death causes the epidermis to separate from the dermis. The syndrome is thought to be a hypersensitivity complex that affects the skin and the mucous membranes. The most well-known causes are certain medications, but the syndrome can also be caused by infections, or more rarely, cancers.

The conditions were first recognized in 1922. A classification was first published in 1933. Children's doctors Albert Mason Stevens and Frank Chambliss Johnson were the ones to discover and document the first case in the *American Journal of Disease*, and the syndrome was subsequently named after these two doctors. There are about 300 cases in the US each year, and 95% of them end with death. The majority of these cases have some or a few of the symptoms—I had them all.

SJS usually begins with a fever, sore throat, and fatigue, which is commonly misdiagnosed and therefore treated with antibiotics. Ulcers and other lesions begin to appear in the mucous membranes, almost always in the mouth and lips, but also in the genital and anal regions. Those in the mouth are usually extremely painful and reduce the ability to eat or drink. Conjunctivitis of the eyes also occurs.

The main cause of SJS is medications. A leading cause appears to be the use of antibiotics, particularly sulfa drugs. Between 100 and 200 different drugs may be associated with SJS. No reliable test exists to establish a link between a particular drug and an individual case of SJS.

Medications that have traditionally been known to lead to SJS, erythema multiforme, and toxic epidermal necrolysis include: sulfonamide antibiotics, penicillin antibiotics, cefixime (antibiotic), barbiturates (sedatives), lamotrigine, Phenytoin (anticonvulsants, e.g., Dilantin), and trimethoprim. Combining lamotrigine with sodium valproate increases the risk of SJS.

Part Two

FEELING ILL

There have been so many warnings to Andre and me to stay covered by the blood and to stay prayed up! What does this mean? Why have we heard this from so many people and so many times within the past three weeks? We pray together, we now study together, and we sit up in bed and have our own bible study together. So why the warnings?

September 3, 2015 was my fifty-seventh birthday! We had just blown out the candles when we got a call that the girls' grandfather had passed away to be with the Lord. The night stopped abruptly. Everything changed; there was no more life in the house. Andre went from person to person holding us, hugging us, loving us. Then, as we dried our eyes, we realized we had to let Amari, my nine-year-old granddaughter, know what had just happened. We just looked at each other for a moment, and then we went in the bedroom and cried and talked, and I decided I would be the one to tell her, but we would sit in the room together. Amari cried and left the room after we all gave her a hug. She then went back in the living room with Andre and he held her on his lap as she cried. He held her tight in his loving arms as she cried until she finally came to grips with the situation. Genesis, miss three-year-old with lots of energy, walked around looking at everyone like, *Come on, guys. Let's continue to have fun, let's sing happy birthday to Mom Mom!* But the night was already done!

†††

Oh my goodness I had a toothache. I wasn't able to go to the dentist until September 10, 2015, and on that day I got there an hour early because I was in so much pain! I was hoping someone had cancelled and they might be able to see me sooner. No such luck! When the dentist finally examined me, he said he would have to refer me to a specialist because I needed a root canal on two of my teeth, and he could not perform the process. He gave me a prescription for penicillin to take for a week to get the infection out so the specialist could do the root canal. I had to wait until September 25, 2015 to have this done.

†††

The next day, September 11, 2015, was my church's Fresh Market event. We gave fresh vegetables, bread, and sweets to the community. I had prayer with our members and gave instructions as directed by our Pastor, Dalyn L. Dunn. But man, my tooth was killing me. I had not eaten anything, so I knew not to take the pills yet. One of our members got me some chicken and mashed potatoes. I could not eat the chicken but I was able to eat the mashed potatoes. I took my first pill. Later I ate another cup of mashed potatoes and took another pill, as instructed. I still was feeling weak and sick because for a week I had not been able to eat anything except applesauce. I told a few members that I wasn't feeling well, and everyone told me it was because I needed to eat something. What they didn't understand was that I had eaten the only thing I could eat, which was the mashed potatoes. Still, the pain was getting worse and I started to feel sick to my stomach! I started thinking to myself, *Are you serious! I have too much to do. This is a major weekend and it is not the time to be sick!*

At this point, I was so weak and sick that I kept asking God to walk and talk for me because I was done! I was tired and then had to deal with, let's just say, some special attitudes. But you know what? Because of how I was feeling, I didn't tolerate anything that was not in order according to Pastor Dunn. In other words, God was moving and walking and talking for me because I stayed in the spiritual, respectful tone, but had no time for anyone out of order!

As the end of the day neared, I told everyone I was going to leave since Pastor Dunn had got there, and due to the fact that Saturday was our community event—called E.P.I.C.—for which I had to make macaroni salad. I also had to cook baked chicken for one of our members and one of my best friends. I needed to be able to host her wedding reception and help out where needed. But as I approached everyone, they all said the same thing: "You need to eat something!" I just looked at everyone because I had eaten what I could! What was wrong with me? Why was I feeling so weak and sick? Why was nobody listening to me when I told them I did eat what I could?

✝✝✝

I finally made it home! It took every bit of energy to make all that salad, but I was able to clean and put the chicken together and let it slow cook in the oven overnight! Praise God I made it through the day! I was so happy to lay down! We had to be back at church at 8:00 a.m. so we could clean the church and get things set up for E.P.I.C.

Part Three
TOO WEAK

Saturday September 12, 2015 was finally here, and so was E.P.I.C., which stands for East Peace In the Community. Yeah! It was finally time for our community event. Super old-school fun! Free food, games, bounce house, and a grilling contest between Pastor Dunn and one of the Deacons. It was scheduled to be an awesome day! But when I opened my eyes I still felt sick! Andre wanted me to stay home. I wanted to, but there was no way I could because of all the events of the day. I also had so much stuff and food I needed to get to the church, and to the wedding reception. Andre was so concerned, but I just moved slow and took my time. We loaded the truck and started on our way. I thought, *If I get something to eat and a 7UP or Sprite, also take no pills today, then maybe I will make it through the day!* So I asked Andre to stop at McDonald's to get me something to eat and drink. Well to my surprise, as soon as I smelled that food I had to open the window because I felt like I was going to get sick! Oh no, I couldn't even drink the Sprite! I started praying, *Please God, not now, please!* I had no energy at all. I started wondering what was going on because I could always drink a Sprite or 7UP and it would calm my stomach a little, but I was even having trouble swallowing the drink. We finally made it to the church, and I gave the food away quickly because I didn't want to see it or smell it. Little did I know the process of poison contaminating my system had already started.

As our members came in to set up they asked me if I was OK. I advised them I still wasn't feeling well, and told them I thought it was the medication. Everyone gave me the same answer, "You have to eat with the medication."

I gave them all the same answer, "I didn't take any medication today and I can't eat because I can't swallow, and even if I could, my stomach is upset!"

But the same thing was repeated all day like no one had heard me: "You have to eat, you have to eat, and you have to eat!" I started to look at everyone with disgust, and wondered why no one was hearing what I was saying!

I started thinking to myself, *I am not stupid enough to take medication without eating, but there is something strange going on with me right now! I will call my family doctor and get him to help me out.* I needed to go to the store and pick up a few things; Pastor Dunn needed another grill, so it would be a good time for me to get some fresh air. Pastor Dunn and Andre left to get the grill and I went to the store. I had a few stops to make. I stopped to see a friend from work who had just started doing nails; her shop was by Kroger where I had to go. Still feeling sick, I had to sit in the car to get enough strength to go inside and get what I needed. Everyone was calling to see where I was, so I finally advised them what I was doing and told them I would be back at the church shortly. Andre wanted to come get me, but I assured him I could make it back. I also had to stop at another friend's house to pick up some watermelon salsa for the reception, which was two minutes away from the church.

†††

I finally made it back to the church! Andre was waiting outside for me, and he asked if I wanted him to drive me to the back parking lot to park the truck. I told him yes, because by that time I was super weak. He then had a few people help me into the church and into my office. I had just enough energy to sit at my desk and hold my head back, trying not to get sick and trying to relax. At this point I was crying a little. Andre came in the office urging me to go home and rest! I was still being hardheaded—saying no because I still had to host the wedding reception and had so much to do at the community event.

First Lady Dunn came into the office, and Andre told her the situation. She gave me the First Lady whipping and told me I was going home, and that she would get someone to handle everything I needed to have done—even the hosting of the reception! Andre called our friend who was having the reception and let them know I was too sick to attend and that we had someone taking our place and bringing the baked chicken and watermelon salsa. Andre then looked at me and said, "Now why didn't you listen to me? It took First Lady to get your butt to go home!"

I told him he was right, smiled and said, "Let's at least buy a plate from the grill-off to take with us, even though I know I won't be able to eat mine." I just wanted to support our church! We finally made it home and I slept all day and all night.

✝✝✝

Sunday morning, I was again not feeling well. Andre wanted me to stay home. But I just pressed my way to church and I promised him I would take it easy. I advised him that because of how I was feeling I needed to be in the house of God so I could feel the spirit on me. I had an easy lesson for the children since it was Pastor Dunn's anniversary.

By the time we got to church, there was no way of faking it; you could tell I still wasn't myself. I managed to make it upstairs for praise and worship. I was only able to sit with the kids and listen to the singing and praising, instead of joining in as I normally do for praise and worship. I sent the kids down to the altar for prayer and I sat at my seat and prayed. We made it back downstairs; I gave a short lesson to the kids. We talked about Pastor's anniversary, and then I advised the kids we were going to make cards for Pastor Dunn. The kids did such an awesome job! I was so proud of them! They really put their hearts into the cards and they could not wait to give them to Pastor Dunn!

As for me, I still could not eat or drink anything. One of the mothers of the church who knew about my history with Sprite and 7UP kept trying to get me to drink the 7UP that I had been trying to drink all morning, but I could still not get it down. One of the other mothers stated that I was not looking well, and the other one was very concerned. As I stood in the middle of the floor looking at the kids, I felt my heart beating to an unbalanced beat, and then it started to tighten up just a little. It wasn't enough to scare me, but I did get light-headed, so I sat down thinking I was doing too much. I sat quiet for about ten minutes and just enjoyed watching everyone. Then I thought, *OK, God, what is really going on with me? This stuff is not normal.*

✝✝✝

Church was finally over so I sent the kids upstairs to their parents. I looked at Pastor Dunn when he came downstairs and advised him that we would not be able to stay for his anniversary service at 5:00 p.m. I knew he wanted us to be there, and my heart ached as I looked in his eyes. It broke my heart when he replied, "Are you sure you guys can't be here?" and I sadly advised him that I was still not feeling well, and that I really needed to go home and get in bed. He then advised us to take it easy and for me to get some rest.

Part Four

WHAT A RIDE

The family was so hungry! Amari was begging, "Mom I am starving! Can we stop and get some Chipotle?" I told her that we would stop on the way home at the one near our house. I had to run upstairs in the sanctuary for a second before we left. One of the ministers asked to speak with me. She told me she had a message from God. She began to tell me how much my husband loves me.

I looked at her and said, "God didn't need to tell you that for me because I know how much my husband loves me!"

She then said, "You don't listen to him or do right by him."

I looked at her and asked, "What are you talking about? I do right by him, and I love him, and we do for each other all the time."

She said, "See! Look at you right now! If he tells you not to worry, you still worry! There are things you just don't do!"

I thought to myself, *Is it me?* Then I thought, *Heck no! I know how much I do, not only for my husband, but for my family and church family also!*

Then she advised me that I had rejected what the doctors had told me! "Look at yourself," she said. "You used to be happy, you had the spirit in your eyes, and you were losing weight! If you don't watch out you will cause yourself to go backward!"

She continued by telling me that this was a problem and that I took on the problems of others. "You're not their dumping ground!" she said. She told me to tell her if she was wrong.

I looked at her in dismay and said, "Actually I am tired of some people!" Little did she know that I meant everyone! No one heard me and no one was listening to me. So I looked at her and told her she was wrong. I knew what she was referring to when she said I had rejected the doctor—it was about my diabetes—but this time it was not about anything other than the medication. Don't get me wrong, she was normally correct. But not this time! So, *NO*, once again I said, "God has spoken to me and it was the medication! Nothing else." I then got enough strength in me and said, "Goodbye," and went downstairs to get my family. As we walked to the truck I thought, *What's wrong with them? What's wrong with them all? Why is it so hard to hear me? Am I speaking a foreign language?* I had to get out of there!

We got in the car to go our usual way home, down Seltzer Rd. to 270 West. Nope! There was an accident on the freeway and it was shut down, therefore we had to find another way home. I thought, *Are you serious? OK, let's take Hamilton Road.* We went to Hamilton Road and it was all backed up and almost at a complete standstill. I thought maybe this was because the freeway was shut down. I started thinking, *God, what is really going on today?* This was totally unreal!

We stopped because the light had changed, and as we looked to the right of us a girl on her motorcycle just fell over on her bike—she laid there motionless! We were in this long line of traffic, and everyone stopped, jumped out of their cars and ran to the girl! They got the bike off of her, but she was still not moving. Someone called 911. I mean, she just fell over in slow motion like

Tim Conway on the *Carol Burnett Show* when he played the old man on the tricycle who falls over in slow motion. That was exactly how this looked. But, after about twenty-five minutes, we looked at each other like, *Here we are, stuck again!*

While we were waiting for the fire truck and ambulance to arrive, I turned and looked at my family and said, "What is really going on today? Is God trying to tell us we should have stayed at church even though I was sick?"

Andre said, "I'm not going to feel bad because you are very sick and we are going to get you home."

Amari said, "I'm so hungry, and I can hardly stand it!"

Lisa said, "Mom, we are going home. We are just stuck."

Finally, at about 5:00 p.m., we made it to our side of town. It took us about three hours to get home, a drive that normally took about thirty-five minutes. We stopped at Chipotle, and fifteen minutes later we were finally walking in our front door. I thought maybe I could eat a small amount because the burrito was soft. Nope! I took one bite and looked at Lisa and said, "Oh my goodness, I am so ready for something but I can't eat this either. Will you eat this for me tomorrow?" That burrito had cost too much to just throw it away after one bite. She agreed!

Part Five
THE POISON

Monday morning I was so excited because I was going to my family doctor! I explained to the doctor what was going on with my tooth and my stomach. I asked him for something that would get the infection out—something that was like the Z-Pak that I was used to taking—but also something to calm my stomach. He gave me Clindamycin (150 mg) to take for fifteen days for the infection, and Ondansetron (4 mg) for my stomach. I was so happy and I got them filled immediately. I was so ready to eat, and Andre and I had not gone out for my birthday meal, so I called him and asked him to meet me at Max & Erma's. He agreed! All of a sudden the wind started blowing; rain was coming down so hard I could not see what was in front of me! Dublin had done construction on my usual route home, I had no idea where I was, and I could hardly see! I took my phone out to MapQuest my way to Max & Erma's. Finally I found a familiar landmark and I knew where I was—thank you, Lord! Andre called and asked if we wanted to cancel because he had been sitting there for about fifteen minutes and it was looking like tornado weather where he was, but since I was finally right across the street, I wanted to go in any way.

There were only about three other couples in the entire restaurant. We had a great time even though I could not eat most of my food. By the time we got home our grill and chairs were turned over, on the other side of our pond there were firetrucks and a rescue truck, and we could see the rental staff and the maintenance men running around. We looked at each other and said, "Wow, what a night! Let's turn in!" That was exactly what we did.

†††

Wednesday I was still feeling sick, but I could eat a small snack-size cup of applesauce and I could drink a cup of water. To me, that was major! I met Andre at bible study and it was great as always. After we had prayer one of Pastor Dunn's godmothers asked me how I was doing. I told her I was still weak and sick. She hugged me and advised me that God was so happy with me and to wait until I saw where He was going to take me next! I cried and told her that I received what she was saying. Little did I know about the real events God was going to take me through. Nothing could have prepared me for these life-changing events!

†††

I kept feeling sick, so that Sunday I stopped taking all of my medication. Monday, September 21, 2015, I woke up feeling a little weaker than before. Andre asked if I was going to stay home. But once again, I pressed my way on to work. *I'm so tired of the small paychecks*, I thought. *I just need to make it until Friday for the root canal.* Throughout the entire day, I felt sick and I could not even finish my applesauce, nor could I get more than a ½ cup of water down. Toward the end of the day, I had trouble focusing on the calls. Finally it hit me! I had to get off the phones because I was going to be sick! I instant messaged my supervisor, left the caller on the phone—my supervisor had to finish the call for me—and I ran to the restroom! After leaving the restroom, I had to go sit in one of the conference rooms to try to get myself together. I tried four times to get the strength to get up and go back to the phones. Finally, I was able to make it, very slowly and carefully. *Thank you, Lord!* I thought.

After I signed back on the phones, my supervisor asked me, "Are you OK?"

I advised her no! I told her that I was going to make it because I was so tired of getting small paychecks.

Two of my coworkers asked, "Ms. Michele are you OK over there? You are very quiet."

I told them no, that I was feeling really, really sick. Praise God, I made it through the day! It was finally over; it was 6:30 p.m.! I called Andre to let him know I was on my way home. I got sick every fifteen minutes like clockwork that night! It had now been four weeks with hardly anything to eat, so I wasn't sure why I was still sick! It had also been a few days since I had any medication.

✝✝✝

September 22, 2015, the next day, I was so weak and tired of being up all night that I could hardly sit on the side of the bed. How could I be this sick with stuff coming out of me when I'd had no food or anything to drink! I looked at Andre and told him I was staying home. He told me that God had woken him up three times that night. The first time, Andre was in this house and he came against demons, but they just burst because of his presence. The second time, God sent him back into the house, and as he walked into each room he would see dead people. But as he entered the rooms they would get up and come back to life! The third time, God told him to pray over me! So he got up and started praying! As he touched me and prayed over me his entire arm felt like fire!

I looked at him and said, "I felt something being pulled out of me but I didn't know what it was!" All of a sudden I stopped getting sick! I looked at him in disbelief and total amazement! This really happened! "Oh my God! Thank you! He pulled that demon out of me!"

Andre kissed me and said, "Call me if you need me." He left for work and I felt peaceful and hoped I would get some rest.

Part Six

HAVE FAITH

†††

My oldest daughter, Lisa, has Multiple Sclerosis. She got that in the Navy. They woke her up the weekend before 9-11 and told her that if they didn't get her out right at that time, she wouldn't be able to get home. The military knew something was about to happen, they just didn't know what! She was stationed in Atsugi, Japan. Her aircraft carrier was the USS Kitty Hawk. They were the first carrier launched after the 9-11 attack.

†††

Andre, Lisa, Amari, and I lived together so we could help Lisa with her daily life routines. She had the master bedroom because it was on the first floor and she could not walk up and down the stairs very well. However, on this day she kept coming upstairs to check on me because I could not do too much of anything but sleep. She tried to get me to eat something but that didn't work. I couldn't swallow anything like food, even the applesauce at this point! I asked her to bring up a cup of ice water. I thought maybe I could drink cold water all day and it would help my stomach feel better. No, I could only take a sip of water every so many hours. After a couple of hours had gone by, I was back in the bathroom getting sick! Finally, about 5:00 p.m., I was able to sleep the rest of the day and night!

✝✝✝

On September 23, 2015, Andre got ready for work and I looked at him even weaker than the day before. I felt so cold! I thought I was getting a cold on top of everything. That would explain why I was so sick. I was afraid to take anything at this point! But even if I could take something I couldn't swallow. I had to think, *Almost four weeks ago I took four penicillin pills, last week I took Clindamycin for six days, I couldn't even make the fifteen-day requirement on that drug and now I am getting a cold! I took an ibuprofen (800 mg) about three days ago. Man I am in bad shape! But to God be the glory that I stopped taking everything on Sunday, so now maybe I will start to feel better!*

Later that afternoon, Lisa came upstairs and advised me that Andre didn't have to pick up Amari from the bus stop. She and her grandmother were going to do it because they were going over to their grandmother's house since they had family in town. They were going to hang out for the day. I advised her to text Andre and I laid back down. Just before it was time for Lisa to leave, she came back upstairs and asked if I needed anything. I said, "Well I finally stopped getting sick, so I will force down a cup of applesauce and try to drink a full cup of water."

Lisa left and I prayed, "Lord I don't need anyone telling me what's wrong with me but You! No one from the church, no messengers, no one from the job, Lord just You! I need a touch from You, Lord! TELL ME WHAT TO DO, LORD. SHOW ME IN YOUR SPIRIT! HELP ME, LORD, RIGHT NOW!" I thought, *I don't want anyone but You, Lord!* He put in my spirit to take a couple of sips of water and to force down a few spoonfuls of applesauce. I did, and then I fell asleep.

WHO COULD HAVE IMAGINED!

I heard the bathroom door open, it was Andre. He asked from the bathroom, "Are you OK, honey?" He told me that he had just seen Lisa and her grandmother at the bus stop. He said, "She sent me three texts, but I didn't get the first one, which told me I didn't have to come home. But something told me to come to the house and check on you since I was already here." He asked if I gotten sick today.

I said, "No, but I still feel really sick to my stomach." I sat on the side of the bed with my back toward the bathroom.

Andre came out of the bathroom and yelled, "OH MY GOD, HONEY! Your skin has turned totally black! I need to call nine-one-one or we need to rush you to the ER!" He then touched my back and my skin peeled off like he had just peeled a banana. Andre yelled even more, "OH MY GOD! What is going on? Let me help you get dressed!" He helped me put some clothes on; I couldn't do too much to my hair, nor did I even think to look in a mirror to see what he was talking about.

We made it slowly to the truck. We had been to the emergency room so many times that we could get there with our eyes closed! But on this day, we got lost! I said in my mind, *Satan is a liar and he will not stop us!* We finally got to the ER. I looked at Andre and said, "Honey I can't hardly walk, I will need a wheelchair. I'm sorry, I just don't have the strength to walk inside." Andre pulled in front of the doors, got a wheelchair and registered me. He also had them give me a bag in case I got sick because I was starting to feel nauseated due to all the moving around. I didn't realize it, but my life had changed at that moment and I would never be the same!

Who could have imagined! What was so funny was that as we were trying to get help, I never saw what I looked like, and Andre tried so hard to stay calm. People stared at me but I didn't give it a second thought! Andre looked at me and said, "You are not coming back home with me because they are going to keep you."

I said, "I know, God showed me also. I am going in, but I am not coming back home today."

What did that mean? God said, "I have you and I am going to change your life. You are going to the next level. You will be new—I love you and you are My child!"

I said, "OK, God! I just need one touch from You, Lord! One touch from You!"

The nurse called my name, and after one look at me she got on the walkie-talkie and said, "We are going to need a bed!" She looked at us and said, "Oh my God! We need to get you in a bed right away!" They got a bed and hooked me up to four bags of IV. They asked what I had been taking and I was able to provide the dates of the penicillin. I had Lisa send me a snapshot of the Clindamycin because I wasn't sure of the name. I also advised them about the ibuprofen 800, and let them know I had not taken anything within the past three days. The doctors checked me out and were all in amazement! I looked at them like, *What is going on?* Finally, they all came in the room and told me they would have to transfer me to Riverside or OSU. They were unable to handle my situation there because I needed to be transferred to the burn unit. We were in shock! The other doctors wanted to send me home with new medications and insisted that I just had an allergic reaction to medication, but the nurse would not let them. She kept pushing them not to release me because she felt like there was more to this. If it were not for her gut feelings, I would have died that night for sure! But God!

Andre contacted Pastor Dunn. He wanted to come to the ER right then, but since we did not know where I was going, we asked him to wait. We contacted the girls and they were concerned! We called Mom in Philadelphia and she wanted to rush up, but we asked her to wait until we found out more information. Something tried to keep us from getting to the hospital in time, but God had other plans for us! My husband had been praying so hard for me, and if he had not been, I would not be here today to tell this story! Thank you, God, for Your loving arms and Your direction in our lives! Andre followed the ambulance as it transported me to OSU Hospital.

Part Seven

THE DISCOVERY

I was finally at the OSU burn unit at 12:16 a.m. on September 24, 2015. So many doctors came in at one time! They asked questions; they moved me around like I was a celebrity! The head doctor said, "We have all studied about what you have but we have never actually seen a real case!"

I asked, "Well, am I going to live?" I looked over at Andre and he had tears in his eyes because he had just seen a few doctors shaking their heads. I thought I heard Andre pleading with God not to take me away from him.

Then the doctor looked at me with a serious look and said, "Let's just say this is very serious. We don't know what will happen. What you have is called Stevens-Johnson Syndrome. You are burning throughout your entire body from the inside out, and it seems to be getting worse. We are going to try to control the situation." They went on to explain that my face was swollen and getting worse, my skin was now peeling and blistering on my back where Andre had touched me, I had conjunctiva drainage, mouth sores, and crusted purulent lips. My eyes were full of mucous and I had a fever. The bottom line was this—I was on fire from the inside of my body and it was moving at a rapid pace, and they had to put the fire out before it killed me, and they had to work quickly!

WHO COULD HAVE IMAGINED!

All at once, just that quick, in a matter of a few hours my entire body was overtaken by a fever, sore throat, nausea, vomiting, abdominal pain, a rash, a headache, my right and left eyes exhibited a discharge, my skin was warm and dry, the rash was macular, there was blistering, burning, itchiness, painful redness on my back that made it hurt just to exist on the bed, my mouth and lips started to drain and bleed, and to go to the bathroom was like fire coming out of me so they gave me a catheter. My blood pressure and sugar were out of control, and my kidneys were failing. In short, my body was preparing to die quickly! I just kept thinking, *Lord just one touch from You! That's all I need, just one touch from You, Lord! This is taking my body; I will not let it take my mind! I refuse to take my mind off of You, Lord! I just need You, Lord!*

Andre had to keep wiping my eyes because they kept crusting up, and it was becoming harder and harder to see. As the doctors talked to each other I heard one say, "Her attitude is so calm and normal through all of this! She is able to communicate with us in such a calming way!" I had seen how afraid they were to touch me. I had Jesus and I knew He would guide me and keep me alert. But the truth was that every touch was filled with unbelievable pain! By the time they got me to my room in the ICU department I could no longer see.

When we were alone, I asked Andre to get a rag and wipe my eyes. He did, and he asked me to try to open them. I did and he asked me, "What can you see?"

I said, "I can't see anything."

He came closer and looked in my eyes and said, "Honey, there is a film over them like a blind person would have."

I didn't know at the time how upset he was because he just walked over to the window and started praying. I thought, *Let me try to open my eyes again.* Oh my God, I saw it! This beautiful Light! I started to walk toward it. It was so bright and beautiful! I put my hands out to touch it, but I couldn't. It was in front of me, then it wrapped all around me, so warm. I spoke with it about my blood pressure, which was 205 over 101. I saw my sugar and it was 162, and I saw my kidneys struggling to maintain. It was like I was watching a movie, looking at all the machines. I started talking and we decided that they would be OK and would get better. I had no worries and again the light became warmer and it seemed to get closer to me, it seemed to hug me. I said in a whisper, "Thank you and I love you!"

Andre came over and asked, "Did you just say something?"

I asked him if I had just been talking to him. He advised me I hadn't because he had been across the room by the window. He said, "Honey your eyes are open, what do you see?"

I said, "Nothing but this beautiful light! Honey, it's so beautiful!" Then I closed my eyes and tried to fall asleep. But this light wouldn't let me, because it was still so bright! Even though my eyelids were closed I could still see it! It seemed like it wrapped itself around me. I no longer felt cold. The light kept me calm and warm.

✝✝✝

Who could have imagined the fight the doctors had on their hands to keep me alive. No one but the blood of Jesus! They had to save my life! In their eyes, it was almost impossible. They told me that they had studied and read about Stevens-Johnson Syndrome, but they had never seen an actual case! The problems that I had were as follows: Toxic epidermal necrolysis (695.15 ICD-9), conjunctivitis in mucocutaneous disease (372.33 ICD-9), AKI (acute kidney injury) (584.9 ICD-9), accelerated hypertension (401.0 ICD-9), type II or unspecified type diabetes mellitus without mention of complication (250.02 ICD-9), and all vitals were uncontrolled, so the fight was on!

The following section is for anyone in the medical field, or those interested in a more technical description of the symptoms I faced. They gave me an ophthalmology exam—for my eyes. My external body showed the extensive SJS erythematous desquamated rash on my face, chest, arms, and skin sloughing on my back. Lids/lashes—right/left showed erythematous peeling rash, mild MGD; scant white mucous, which discharged at medical canthus, conjunctiva/scleral-melanosis, palpebral conjunctiva without membrane, cornea-clear/tr inf speak, anterior chamber—deep and quiet, iris-round and reactive, lens- tins, vitreous—normal, and mood/affect—normal, fundus exam- right/left was c/d ratio 0.6, macula flat and attached; good flr, and vessels—attenuated.

Part Eight
MEDICATION LIST

In the history of the hospital, they had never given as much medication to one person as they had to give me to keep me alive for this type of case! It was amazing to them. The problem was getting my vitals back to a living state and keeping them under control. The next few pages may not seem like an important read to you, but God is sharing this in hopes that it may help someone else. It is to save the life of anyone else who comes in contact with SJS.

They gave me:

- Ascorbic acid 250 mg — twice a day — tablets (the highest ever)
- Clobetasol 0.05% ointment — apply to affected areas on the face
- Dapagliflozin Propanediol (Farxiga) 5 mg — one per day
- Docusate 100 mg — one capsule twice a day
- Erythromycin 5 mg/gm ointment — apply thin ribbon inside lower eyelid
- Famotldine 20 mg — one tablet a day
- Hydralazine 25 mg — one tablet every eight hours
- Lidocaine (Xylocaine) 80 ml, alum/mag hydroxsimethicone 80 ml

mouthwash — 15 ml every six hours or as needed

- Hydromorphone (Dilaudid) injection 1 mg — intravenous per day
- Methylprednisolone Sodium Succinate (Solu-medrol) 250 mg in sodium chloride 0.9%, with overfill 64 ml (total volume) IVPB 250 mg — by intravenous every six hours
- Potassium Chloride (K-DUR, Klor-con m20) tablet ER 40 m Eq — two tablets once a day
- Potassium Chloride 10 m Eq in sterile water 100 ml premix IVPB — 100 ml — by intravenous every hour
- Amlodipine (Norvasc) 10 mg — one tablet per day
- Dextrose D50% injection 7.5–25g – 15–50 ml — intravenous as needed for low blood sugar
- Erythromycin (Romycin) Ophthalmic ointment — one application in both eyes at bedtime
- Heparin injection 5.000 units — 1 ml three times a day
- Losartan–Hydrochlorothiazide 100–25 mg — one per day
- Metformin 500 mg — twice per day
- Multivitamin w/minerals (Therapeutic-m) — one per day
- Nifedipine 30 mg tablet SR 24HR — once per day
- Oxycodine 5 mg/5 ml solution (Roxicodone) — take 5–10 ml every three hours or as needed for pain
- Polyethylene glycol (Miralax) 40 mg — one packet by mouth per day or as needed for constipation
- Polyvinyl alcohol — povidone 1.4–0.6% solution — one drop in both eyes four times per day
- Prednisone 20 mg–40 mg — seven doses per day

- Senna 8.6 mg — one per day
- Vitamin A 10,000 units — one per day
- Zinc Sulfate 220 mg — one per day before breakfast
- Hydralazine (Apresoline) 15 mg in sodium chloride 0.9%, with overfill 60.75 ml (total volume) IVPB take 15 mg — intravenous every four hours or as needed to hold high blood pressure (SBP < 160)
- Insulin Lispro (Humalog) injection — by subcutaneous route four times per day with meals and at bedtime
- Labetalol (Normadyne) injection 10 mg–2 ml by intravenous every six hours
- Lactated Ringers IV Solution — intravenous continuous
- Magic mouthwash (standard) — 15 ml by mouth every six hours
- Metoprolol (Lopressor) 5 mg in sodium chloride 0.9%, with overfill 65 ml (total volume) IVPD — by intravenous every six hours or as needed for blood pressure (SBP >170)
- Nifedipine (Procardia XL) tablet XL 30 mg — one per day
- Ondansetron 4 mg/2 ml (Zofran) injection 4 mg–2 ml by intravenous every six hours
- Pantoprazole (Protonix) 40 mg — one per day
- Polyvinyl Alcohol — povidone (Refresh) ophthalmic solution — one drop in both eyes four times a day

There may be some things listed more than once. The reason for this is because the medicines that were selected depended on my vitals. This list is strictly to assist with the medications that might be used to save someone else's life.

Now there was also another problem that I haven't even said too much about. I absolutely hated taking pills! So I had all these pills to take, and on top of it all, I was having problems swallowing! Even worse, when I needed to go to the restroom, I felt like a dragon—only instead of fire coming out of my mouth, I felt like I had fire coming out of my vagina! It felt like pure fire in the restroom!

Part Nine

ARE YOU SURE

The doctors came and told me they had to cut a piece of my skin off because they needed to determine if I had SJS. They had to do a skin biopsy. The presence of full-thickness necrosis of epidermal keratinocytes could be compatible with either Toxic Epidermal Necrolysis or Stevens-Johnson Syndrome. Clinical-pathology correlation would be necessary. The test came back! Now for the assessment and plan! Below are the doctors' findings:

I had Stevens-Johnson Syndrome with ocular findings in both eyes, with associated blepharitis/MGD, mucous-like discharge; no membranes or symblepharons were noted. I was positive for dry eyes and symptoms SPK 0S>0D; no corneal ulcers or infiltrates were noted—cont abx—steroid combo for ocular SJS with Tobradex drop QID and ointment qhs in both eyes, defer systemic treatment of SJS to primary team.

My primary doctor was Dr. Deepak Rai, MD. He signed off in agreement with all the findings. They confirmed that I did not have the flu or the Toxic Epidermal Necrolysis. I had SJS, likely induced by penicillin and/or Clindamycin, which I was taking for dental pain prescribed by the dentist. The hospital notes from my case continue below:

WHO COULD HAVE IMAGINED!

I had dermatology burns, ophthalmology on board (I had conjunctiva involvement as well), AKI—resolved. Etiology likely perennial given poor PO intake and likely volume loss from skin—will stop IVF. Hypertensive urgency with history of HTN—etiology is due to high dose steroids as well as being off home medications, continue steroids at the highest dosage 250 mg three times per day. Back with multiple areas of skin sloughing, with overlying dressing, face with multiple areas of hyper pigmentation/ small areas of sloughing, upper chest with bandage from skin biopsy.

†††

The next morning finally came! They noted no acute events overnight. I was a little down from going through everything, but had good support—Andre and the girls—and pain was much improved. I was able to eat and drink a little. My blood pressure would go from 153/86, then 162/78, and finally down to 142/72. Within minutes my blood pressure would go back up to 194/88. They were having so much trouble trying to maintain my blood pressure and my sugar.

That morning I thought, *OK, Lord! I don't need any more stressed looks from the doctors. They are excited about my case, though. Everyone is coming in to see me like I am a celebrity! But I need You, Lord! Just one touch from You, Lord is all I need! Satan has my body, but I will not surrender my mind! I will keep it totally on You, Lord. Tell me what to do, show me how to help the doctors. Guide me, lead me, Lord. I just need Your touch!*

So God stepped in and showed me! It was like watching a movie.

The notes stated: Mrs. Moore is a 57-year-old female with h/o of HTN, DM who presents with diffuse, painful rash, sloughing skin on lips and back and discharge from eyes. Three weeks ago she was otherwise healthy, but had a tooth pain. She went to her dentist who prescribed penicillin. After two days she started vomiting and had nausea and she stopped taking the penicillin. She was switched to clindamycin and continued taking it for six days. She continued to have vomiting and nausea, but this was common for her whenever she took antibiotics. She has had decreased PO intake for the last three weeks. On Monday (four days ago), she woke up with diffuse rash and she noted peeling of lips and discharge from eyes. She also reports a headache and took Ibuprofen 800 as is her practice. The rash increased over the ensuing days with increasing pain and, on day of admission, husband rubbed her back and the skin sloughed off. She was still reporting vomiting. She was taken to Dublin ER and then transferred to OSU ICU. She was seen by dermatology, burn surgery, and ophthalmology here and started on IV Solumedrol and maintenance IV fluids. She was monitored for continued skin sloughing which did progress. Michele Moore's events from the last 12-24 hours were reviewed. Overnight the patient received an additional PRN Dilaudid for pain. During sleep she was incontinent of urine and we therefore have been unable to measure UOP accurately. She denies any headache, chest pain, shortness of breath. She notes that the initial symptoms of dysphagia are improving, but notes some burning of her lips when she eats.

One major thing they forgot—the stupid tooth no longer hurt!

In the name of Jesus, are you serious! All of this and no toothache! God You do have jokes—that's all I can say! Does this all mean there is a higher message? Show me, Lord—one touch!

Part Ten
VISITORS

I was in my ICU room. I could see a little. But there was a fog over my eyes. Andre looked so tired. He couldn't sleep or eat. He just prayed, and I could hear him say, "Lord don't take my wife from me!"

Pastor Dalyn Dunn wanted to come see me at the Dublin ER room, but we asked him to wait until we knew where I would be. Pastor made it to see me the next day! Even though he tried not to show it, I could see the shock on his face when he saw me. He had prayer over me! I love my Pastor to life! The children came after Pastor Dunn left. Surprisingly, Lisa was OK. She was the main one I worried about because of her Multiple Sclerosis. Amari was very upset that she was not allowed in the ICU. She wanted to see me so bad to make sure I was all right! I looked over and I could see Andre holding Renee. He was trying to make her be strong when she came in the room. But when she walked in the room her body went limp like she was going to faint! She cried out, "Oh my God, Mommy, can I just touch you and give you a hug!" I cried with her as we hugged. I told her that I would be OK. After a moment she had to leave the room. She couldn't take it anymore. I still had not seen what everyone else was seeing. I had just seen the looks on their faces.

While the girls were in the lobby a really good friend from church came to see me. She would not stay away even if you paid her to. We are that close. Her name is Ms. Eula. She was dropped off at the hospital and she was determined to find me! She tried to get Andre to eat, but he was in another state of mind. She sat out in the lobby with Amari, Lisa, Renee, and Marguell, Renee's boyfriend.

Finally, I looked at Andre and the nurse and asked them to help me go to the restroom. I was so weak that I could hardly walk. OH MY GOD! The fire coming out of me just to use the restroom! Then I gently pulled myself up and over to the mirror. For the first time I wanted to take a look at myself. I was shocked! Oh my God! Who was the person looking back at me in the mirror? She looked like a monster! I started to fall to the ground as I cried out loud. Then I asked Andre how he could even stand to look at me! How would he be able to continue to love me? Oh my God! I didn't know I looked like that!

Andre said very calmly, and in the sweetest, most sincere voice, "Honey you look beautiful to me. Calm down, don't worry. I love you. You are so beautiful!"

This was unconditional love. I knew he was not joking or just saying that. He meant it! As he and the nurse helped me back to the bed, I was still crying.

†††

The next day my beautiful First Lady, Dawn Dunn, came to visit me. I love her so much. I saw the tenderness in her eyes as she looked at me. Then God gave me the chance to talk with her one-on-one. I needed to talk with her about what I had been advised that last Sunday I was at church. I wanted clarity on what I was thinking, and she gave me just what I needed as always. She prayed with me and headed on her way. I was so grateful!

†††

The next morning about 7:00 a.m., the desk nurse came in the room and asked if a visitor could come in. Andre and I looked at each other like, *Who is here this early?* It was the minister I had spoken with last Sunday. When the door opened all I could do was cry. I sang, "The devil thought he had me, but he didn't know who my daddy was!"

The minister stayed with us for about four to five hours, I think (I don't remember exactly). All I know is that it was a beautiful visit. She came to say, "I was wrong! You told me it was the medicine and it was! God really did show you!" She really didn't want to leave us. She worried about Andre not eating.

There was something the minister told me on that last Sunday that was true: "Your husband really loves you."

She was right! I thought. He had to really love me to tell me I was beautiful and to be able to look at my face! Thank you, Lord, for putting her in my life!

It was Ohio State game day. The traffic was already there because people had started tailgating as early as 6:00 a.m. After Minister left, two of my good friends from church came to see me. They were mother and daughter. It was Ms. Eula and Linda. They did things to help us out in their own special way! They cleaned things up around me and cut up my food so I could try to swallow it. They made sure we were OK. It was Linda's birthday. To be with me that day made it even more special. Her mom said, "After seeing you, Linda cried all the way home!" Not the normal little cry, the hard, broken-hearted cry! The girls made their way back up to give Andre some food. They had a hard time because of all the OSU traffic. Another set of friends came to see me. It was Deacon Terry and Deaconess Billie Graves. The shock of my appearance was all over their faces. Terry had a hard time looking at me, because it made him so sad. My nephew and his mom, who is one of my best friends, also came to see me. It was Jaylen and Dalene. Dalene took a picture of me to make sure I had it for later. I did ask her not to share it though. The picture showed me three days later, and it was still mild compared to what I had originally looked like.

The doctors came and gave me the good news that I could finally be moved out of ICU and into a regular room. Finally, 9-26-2015, I had a turnaround! They started seeing improvements. My vision started to improve. There was still a cloud over my eyes, but I could see the lights being flashed in my eyes and suddenly my eyes started to clear up and I got a good look at the young lady who had been treating and monitoring me. I looked at her, and in a soft soothing voice said, "Hi! It is so wonderful to open my eyes and see a young, black, beautiful woman taking care of me! I am so happy."

She smiled and blushed and said, "Thank you." She was so young and graceful. At least that was how she looked in this new set of eyes that God had bestowed on me! Even though there was still a fog over my eyes, it was beautiful to see and look around at life! To see my husband, to see the other nurses—it was wonderful. You don't realize how precious things are until you cannot use them properly. Things turned around in small doses, but it was enough to take me out of ICU. I was stable. *Lord I just want to thank You!* I had no doubt and no fear. I had Abraham's faith. You could not tell me that God didn't have His hands wrapped around me! My God was so beautiful and awesome! The doctors were amazed at the turnaround! The doctors told me I would be in the hospital for a few weeks or longer. God had other plans. God gave me a vision that I would be going home soon.

Andre needed to go home and freshen up since he had been there for three days. God put in my spirit to have him bring me our bill folder. He really got concerned and asked if everything was OK. "Are we behind on our bills? What's the problem?" he asked.

I explained that we were not behind, but the Father had my mind and He placed it in me to keep things in order—for He is a God of order—and to not let anything go undone! When Andre and the girls came back, he had everything. The next thing I heard was the doctors saying they still were having trouble with some of my vitals. They were still fighting to get them back in line. I was in a small room with two beds. It was so small! They advised me I would have no roommate so I could spread some of my things around, which made me very happy. The only fear I had was seeing Amari and Genesis. I was afraid that they would be scared of me!

A family friend/daughter had Amari, and Lisa and Renee had Genesis. The thought of Amari and Genesis seeing me like this made me afraid, but they both came running in the room like there was a fire! Genesis, my three-year-old, said, "Mom Mom—you got balloons! Can I play with them?"

While she was hugging me so tight, I laughed and said, "Yes!"

Amari hugged me super tight and said, "I knew you were going to be OK, Mom! I just needed to see you. They wouldn't let me see you! Now I am OK!"

I thought to myself and said out loud, "I love you, Amari!"

That was pretty deep for a nine-year-old. I sat up in the bed and the nurse came in and said, "Mrs. Moore we are having problems with your blood pressure and sugar." Then she stopped and asked, "What are you doing?" I had my bills on the bed and I was writing out checks.

"I have to take care of our household items as I always do," I told her. She laughed! So I advised our family friend, whose name was Mia, what things I needed Lisa to mail so her bills could be in order.

Very concerned, Renee said, "Mom! What are you doing? You are doing bills and not relaxing, that's why your blood pressure was high and everything else is up! You need to relax!"

I looked around at my family and said, "God has given me my orders. If I get this done I can then sit back and relax. He knows my heart." So everyone, including the nurse, let me finish what I was doing. Once I was done, they watched me sit back and I looked so peaceful. They all kissed me and left. Another best friend and her grandson came to visit me. It was Toni! Instead of seeing the shock in her eyes, I saw so much love in her eyes. I love her so much for coming to see me. When they left another best friend who had been in my life for years came to visit. I had not seen her for a long while. It was Zeta. I was so happy to see her, and she gave me some good information about what I was going to have to do, and also about being around others. I slept in peace! Perfect Peace!

†††

Monday morning Renee called crying because she was so upset! She said, "I can't work and I can't bring myself to do anything but cry!" She was so tired in her mind and heart. I advised her that I needed her to be strong. I needed her to handle a few things. I could not get the rest I needed until she started to see things in the way God needed us to see things. I needed her to get up and go to work and try to get back on track with her life. She cried even harder and said, "I will try, Mom." She decided to contact her job and she handled her finances! I was so proud of her! To God be the glory, because everything worked out in her favor! God gave her everything and more; He is so awesome! He worked everything out in His wonderful plan, and we knew it was because of Him. No one could have done the things for us as He did—only God's way works! After that I was able to lay down and go to sleep. Still, my vital signs were off the chart. But I knew it was because of the steroids so I wasn't worried like the doctors were because God had His hand on me! But they were still very worried because they were working hard to get my body organs to function normally, and get them turned around. Pastor David came to visit. I was so happy to see him; we had a wonderful blessed visit! He is Pastor Dalyn Dunn's brother. I love that family to life!

The pain in my back from my skin peeling off was almost unbearable. My mouth and lips hurt and felt like fire was coming out of them because of the peeling skin and the blood and mucous that keep coming out of them. I had to keep cleaning my eyes because of the yellow discharge coming out of them. My heartbeat had a distant sound like it was barely beating. To turn, move, or even sit up in the bed was extremely painful because of the rapid skin rashes and patches where skin was lost, which now populated my arms, butt, upper legs, and back. I had increased denuded blisters on my upper back. As the day continued so did the increased skin loss. They still had to continue to give me steroids and I was still burning on the inside. They had to give me artificial tears because I had none. They gave me magic mouthwash, which numbed the pain on the inside of my mouth. They were concerned about the increase of my skin loss. I kept a fever. There was still vaginal irritation and dysuria felt to be related to sloughing of mucous membranes. They started me on clobetasol cream three times a day. Because I had such a hard time swallowing, I still had a problem with ongoing fluid losses. They had to continue with the IV hydration, MIVF to 200 ml/hr. It was so hard to sleep, but God suddenly woke me up and I started to feel different! I felt like my body was changing.

Part Eleven

THE TURN AROUND

The doctors came in the room in amazement! They looked at me and said, "You are going home tomorrow!"

I yelled, "What!" *Oh, my God, You are so amazing! Oh, my God, You are so wonderful! I love You so much!*

The doctors told me I would be released about 11:00 a.m. or a little later.

I said, "OK!"

I had a hard time sleeping! I wanted to go home so bad. God showed me that within seven days He died and then He rose! I was crucified! But now I live! Because of the lesions on my body, I could not have any tape on any dressing to my skin. My blood pressure went to 171/80.

†††

The next morning, September 30, 2015: Time to go home! They brought in a roommate early that morning. There was a new smell in the room that was making me feel sick to my stomach! I sat up on the side of my bed at 6:00 a.m. Lisa called and told me to relax and sit back. I explained that I needed to get out of there. I was feeling so sick because of this new smell in the room. Breakfast came; I looked at it and could not eat anything! They thought it was because of me not being able to eat again. I asked for nausea medication. It didn't come right away; I was feeling worse so I asked again with urgency! I listened to the nurses trying to keep the other patient calm. I couldn't relax. So much was going on in my head and I had to get out of that room!

Renee called and said, "Mom try to sit back and relax."

I couldn't get off the side of the bed, so I just sat there looking at the television. But one thing was for sure, I was not going to lay back down in that bed! The nurse came in and asked me if they could get me anything. I said, "I just need the doctor to come in and release me!" The nurse came back and advised me that since I was going home, the doctors were tied up with sick patients. They had to take care of them first and they might be tied up with them for awhile. Sometimes the released patients got pushed to the back burner. I didn't care, in my mind someone was coming soon!

I still sat on the side of my bed. Deacon and Deaconess Rayford called and said, "We will be there at eleven o'clock." As I sat in the room, the smell got worse. The nurses came and took the other patient out for a test. I looked around the room and you could hardly move because of all my machines and the other machines for my roommate. It took so much out of me, but I decided to get washed up and dress. I looked at the smallest shower I had ever seen and decided I couldn't even use it. I guess I didn't realize how much energy it would take me to get washed and dressed. I had to sit back down on the side of the bed to rest and get myself together after I got dressed. My roommate was back and her family was there also.

Then there was a beautiful sight! It was the Rayfords! They had just walked in the room. I was so happy to see them. We started putting everything together and in bags. There was nowhere for them to sit, so we just enjoyed talking and being together, me on the side of the bed and them standing at the foot of the bed. They never worried about the time. My lunch was brought in the room. Mashed potatoes and gravy, chicken strips, and an ice-cream cup. Mind you the smell in my room was now making me feel even sicker. But I tried to eat—I took a spoonful of the mashed potatoes and it grossed me out, then I tried the chicken strips, took one bite... No! Gross! My mouth was on fire so I ate the ice-cream cup. Deacon and Deaconess Rayford laughed at my face and said, "We can stop and get you something to eat on the way home."

I looked at them and said, "I can't do this, I need to get out of here. All I wanted was some real food."

The doctor came rushing in the room. He looked at me and said, "Oh my, hold on for one minute. You are really ready to go home. Give me about forty-five minutes to get everything ready."

The nurse came in the room and said, "You can't eat again?" I advised her it was the taste of the food, it was not good. I also advised her that I had a strange smell in my system and it affected the taste of the food. The Rayfords teased and joked with the nurse about the food. The nurse said, "I mostly bring my own lunches."

I looked at everyone and said, "Sister Spencer from church is already at the house. She stayed with me and took care of me when I had my foot surgery, and bless her heart she is going to stay with me and take care of me now." I advised them all that I wanted some real food! I just wanted to get to Sister Spencer and have a peanut butter and jelly sandwich on some real bread—my Sarah Lee Honey Wheat. The doctor came with the medication prescriptions and the release papers. There were so many medication prescriptions and instructions! They had contacted Nightingale Home Healthcare to come and check on me and help me adjust. My appetite was almost back to normal, and I was eating 50–100% of my meals. I was able to chew and swallow. During this time I had lost twelve pounds. To be released I also needed a Nutrition Plan of care which consisted of:

1. Continue current diet order as tolerated (diabetic)
2. Monitor/encourage PO intake
3. Monitor weight status and lab values
4. Continue to follow up on nutrition

The other follow-up instructions were to have follow-up appointments with dermatology, and possibly with ophthalmology.

Part Twelve
HOME

We got in the car and I got in the back seat. Oh my God, I had the balloons in front of me and they smelled like the room! I could not wait to get home and get out of that car! Hallelujah! We made it home! I walked in and was so excited to be home! Lisa and Sister Spencer were so happy to see me! The first thing Sister Spencer asked me was what did I want to eat.

"Yes, you know me well," I said. "A peanut butter and jelly with real bread and a glass of water."

Everyone in the house laughed and said, "OK." Deacon and Deaconess Rayford went to Giant Eagle and got all of the prescriptions filled for me. I enjoyed my sandwich like I was eating a steak and a baked potato. That sandwich was the best, but that night was so hard! My mouth woke me several times. It was unbearable—there was mucous and blood coming out and I cried and I tried to pray the pain away. But nothing worked to ease the pain. I just had to cry it out and let it run its course.

The next morning, since I couldn't sleep, I needed to show Sister Spencer and Lisa how to get to the bank. I also needed some medical supplies that I needed to pick out for myself. I knew I wasn't supposed to go out, but God showed me that I was in His care. So, we covered me up—I put on a hat and gloves, had a blanket, and sunglasses—I had the works. I sat in the back seat very weak, and advised them where to go and how to get there. I knew God was with me, but they could not understand how much. So I shared with them the things I was led to do and they listened and watched. They did not question me.

There was a wig shop next to where Lisa had to go, so I advised Sister Spencer that I needed to go in there and look for a wig. I was very careful; the spirit was with me because the whole store was empty. I didn't have to come into contact with anyone. Then a young lady entered the store. She walked over to me and said, "I've never tried to wear a short wig, so let me try it."

My face was half black, pink, and weird-looking! I looked at her and said, "I never imagined that I would look like this and have to buy a wig." I told her that God was good and I found the wig that looked like me and I slowly made my way to the register. I looked up after I paid for the wig and I saw this bling bling hat that said, "HOPE." I said, "Hope! That's it! May I please have that hat because I really need it right now!" I was so hopeful in my heart, and all of a sudden I felt so pleased!

Lisa was ready just after I got back in the car and we went farther down the street. We needed to stop for medical supplies and food. I said, "I am led to stop at this Save-A-Lot." It was just before the freeway to get back to our side of town. Sister Spencer and Lisa were advising me not to get out of the car again. But I had to go to the restroom. We went into the store and I slowly started looking for someone to ask where the restroom was. The funny thing was, as I looked around in this large store, only about three other people were there as well.

As I was walking my cell phone rang. It was one of the sisters from the church. She didn't realize what I had just gone through. She was going through a lot herself. Her grandson was the one who told her to call me because I was on his mind. I think he was only five years old. After she cried she told me that at church on Sunday, Pastor Dunn had everyone come up to the altar and hold me up in prayer. But when she tried to get up the spirit would not let her, and then she saw this bright light. I told her how I had seen His marvelous light and that was what she was seeing. She cried even harder, and I advised her that no matter what she was going through to keep pressing because God was handling it! I advised her not to stop and to keep trusting because God had put in my spirit that she was going to be OK, and we hung up the phone.

The manager then just walked up to me out of nowhere, so I asked him to direct me to the restroom. Still there was hardly anyone in the store with us. When I opened the door to the restroom, it was amazing! It was so sterile, so clean, so bright that I had to hold my hand up to my face because the light was so bright! I knew right away it was God's light again because it was the same as it had been when I was in the hospital, and I knew that's why that restroom looked like that. I had never seen anything like that before! His protective hand was covering me! Amazing, just amazing!

After I was done, Lisa with her motorized cart, Sister Spencer with her shopping cart, and I were ready to check out. The store manager was behind us again—keep in mind we did have all three carts full of stuff—so he moved the other two customers to another line and had the cashier check only the three of us out. I made sure Sister Spencer and Lisa knew God was with us. When we got home, I was wiped out for the rest of the night.

†††

Now, if you remember, when I thought I was going to die, I asked God for one touch. I spoke with Pastor Dunn that night and he asked me why I kept talking about "one touch." So I explained that I had asked God for this touch to save my life. One Touch! Pastor Dunn said, "I preached Malachi 3:1-4, 'The

WHO COULD HAVE IMAGINED!

Refiner's Touch' on Sunday. We praised God so hard and we knew He was in our midst!"

How could God give me what Pastor's message was? Other spiritual things also happened. I would sleep but the spirit would wake me up and we would talk in tongues! For about two years I had asked God to let me speak in tongues. I used to watch everyone else and I would want it so bad!

†††

October 2, 2015, I had my first visit with the home healthcare nurse. The nurse's name was Reta DiDonato. She was so fabulous! I loved her spirit from the very first time I met her. She walked in and said, "Oh my God! How are you here? I had to research your case because we have studied about Stevens-Johnson Syndrome but we never had an actual case! You should not even be here, let alone home after what you have been through. How is that possible? Only seven days, this is unreal! Your faith is what kept you, and you truly are a walking miracle! You need to document this and make the public aware of the dangers of the medication as well as the SJS."

I told her that God had placed it in my heart to do just that—to document this event. She just lifted her hands in the air and said, "Thank God for you! There is truly a God! You will be an inspiration to others." I felt like crying because seeing and hearing about the pain I was in all night, every night, made her feel so bad. We had a great visit.

†††

The next couple of days were very strange. Everything we watched on TV had a strange spiritual meaning—old TV shows like *Daniel Boone*, *Perry Mason*, *Andy Griffith*, weird old movies, and even *The Smurfs*. I felt like I was living in a twilight zone!

Saturday my best friends came over again (Ms. Eula and Linda). They came so Ms. Eula could make me her famous chicken spaghetti. My cartoon buddy and best friend (Linda) and I sat and watched cartoon movies. We watched *Tom and Jerry* with the magic dragon, and then we watched *Brave*. They were both great movies, but once again both had spiritual meanings. I needed to see my little granddaughter Genesis. I was feeling the need. She came over just before the ladies left. God put in my spirit to anoint her head and to braid it in a certain way. Then on Sunday God had me do the same thing to Amari. It was strange but true and spiritual. In everything and everywhere I looked I saw spiritual things.

Sunday I told Andre that I needed to get out of the house. He and Lisa took me to Wal-Mart and I agreed to stay in the truck. I was just sitting there and this couple came up to that truck and just walked around it, I mean walking around it trying to look inside, just admiring it. I just sat there listening to gospel music on my cell phone, just crying and praising God! Lisa and Andre came out of the store and said, "Some strange things are happening!" They said this couple had been watching them so hard they ran their cart into the wall. Lisa laughed at them. Then, as they went to the checkout line, Andre turned around to say something to them, but the couple would not even look at them. In fact, they would not let their cart or themselves get close to Lisa and Andre, so there was this big gap between them and the couple in the checkout line.

Andre said, "It was like they were afraid to be close to us." I explained to them that there was a spiritual warfare going on right at that moment with our family. The Lord saved my life and Satan was not happy because I still didn't turn my back on God! I am like a Jobette! He stole my body but he couldn't steal my mind because it stayed on Jesus! The couple they saw in the store was an evil spirit, and after seeing it, they started seeing things with different eyes. We got back home and enjoyed the rest of our day. That night, dreams, talking in tongues, it just took over my body—I was sweating, and then the pain, I couldn't take it! I'd cry, I'd beat my legs, I begged God to please help me! It was a rough, rough night!

Monday we had another great meeting with Reta. She was very concerned that I was still in so much pain. She started reviewing my pain medication notes, but to her things didn't add up. She advised that she would check things out. And she did! I had no good pain medication. She left messages for Dr. Schumacher and others. Finally, at about 8:00 p.m., we got the call that one of the doctors had called in a prescription for Oxycodone. Andre came home with a beautiful card.

But once again he was met with another spirit. He was at Kroger and had already checked out and was waiting on his two coworkers to get checked out. There was a cashier all the way on the other side of the checkout register lanes, which was not even near Andre, who had at least fifteen people in his line because the store was so crowded. This cashier turned around and did a double look at Andre and actually yelled across the room at him, "Hey! Are you being helped?" He was so loud and out of order that even the cashier who had waited on Andre turned around and looked at him like he was crazy. Andre's coworker checked out and told Andre that it was strange, but to just let it go. They got in the truck and had to agree again that it was really strange! When he got home the card had scriptures on it and it was very Godly. I explained that once again he'd had an encounter with a spirit. How dare he not only save my life, but now he has the audacity to bring me a Godly card! How dare he!

We enjoyed the rest of the night. But that evening, pain and dreams again! God had put in my spirit that when I was speaking in tongues I was speaking in a different language, and that no one at church would be able to interpret it because it came from Him and was between Him and me. Then He put in my spirit that His ways were not our ways, and His time was not our time. He said that everything would work out for our church. We were renting the church but there were people who were not from the USA trying to take it from us because they wanted the back bingo hall. As a small church we were just trying to hold on!

Our church is so good for the community. We have fresh produce giveaways once a month, we try to help everyone we can, but mostly we are family with each other! These strangers wanted to take our church from us so they could continue to use the bingo hall for their receptions!

Tuesday I got medication for my pain. That morning God had me anoint Sister Spencer's head and then Lisa's head. Once again He had me braid it in a certain way! Several people from the church brought food to us during this time, and Deaconess Rayford took me to my appointments so Sister Spencer could pick up Amari from the bus stop.

Early Wednesday morning God got me up with the pain and put in my spirit to lean not onto my own understanding, but to lean onto His understanding and not to question anything. Then about 4:00 a.m. He showed me some gifts for three couples who were getting married. It was strange because the items for them really had meaning that spoke in their lives. I know this because after speaking with one couple, they really truly appreciated the gift and loved it, and it also meant something to them.

Later, Reta came and Sister Spencer explained that I finally had the pain medicine, but my lips and mouth were still on fire and discharging blood and mucous at night. Once again Reta got on the phone. "There must be something that can be done," she explained. It was later that night when she called back with one of the doctors on the line. The doctor needed my pharmacy information, and called in a tube of Lidocaine ointment which actually numbed my tongue and lips. Even though I hurt, it was now manageable. It was nothing like it was. I still woke up that night, but it was not as bad.

Thursday Pastor Dunn called, and I found out that once again what God had put in my spirit two nights ago about His understanding and His ways not being ours is what Pastor taught for bible study. Once again, we knew God was in our midst! There was no way I could have known what Pastor Dunn had taught about that night! Glory to His Name!

Friday was Reta's last day with me. She was going to another agency. We had a great visit. Sunday morning at 5:00 a.m. God woke me up and put in my spirit to dance for the church. They were to go to Indianapolis for the second service. We could not get the bus this year so everyone going would have to drive their own cars. Because of financial issues, the only ones driving and going were Pastor Dunn, First Lady—they would drive their other car—and Deacon and Deaconess Rayford.

The song "This is War" came on! I danced with everything in me, even though I was still very weak. Sister Spencer was up and she just laughed and smiled and enjoyed it. Then we ate breakfast around 7:00 a.m. After all of that I was so tired that I slept from 8:00 a.m. until 2:00 p.m.

When I finally woke up I had a missed call from Deaconess Rayford. I returned her call. She said, "I called to tell you about a blessing!"

She told me they were getting ready to leave when Deacon Terry came running back into the church and said, "There is a bus out there!"

Pastor Dunn and Deaconess Rayford were like, "No way! There can't be because we didn't order one!" They looked at the receipt and it just stated, "Paid." There were no names, nothing except paid.

Deaconess Rayford said, "I asked the bus driver if he was sure the bus was for us."

The driver said, "Yes, I am here to take all of you to Indianapolis and the bus is paid in full."

All I could do was cry and thank God! I told her how God had me get up and dance for them.

Pastor said, "I don't know how, but I'm not going to question God, and so many of our members get to go out of town!"

God is awesome. For most of the day I cried for them in amazement.

Monday came and Reta came! She released me that day from home healthcare. I was able to start going outside without my mask, and she said I could go to church in a couple of weeks. She also wanted me to try to walk more and get out of the house. Maybe go to the mall. I was so excited! I knew it would be hard because it still took a lot out of me to move around, but I also knew I would be OK because God had me. Maybe one day we could take a family trip and include Sister Spencer. Maybe God would help us save our church. Andre and I never had a real honeymoon, so maybe that would also happen one day.

I don't know what God has in store for us, but I know He is real and He lives in my family (which includes Sister Spencer) and me! I AM SO THANKFUL THAT HE SPARED ME AND DECIDED TO SAVE MY LIFE! Hallelujah to His Name!

Part Thirteen
THE CONCLUSION

What did I want out of this book? I needed to let everyone who is willing to read this know that you *can* survive from Stevens-Johnson Syndrome. It will be a fight. But know that blood clots can form within eight weeks. There are warnings to all medications. You must watch closely for small signs. Nothing is normal. Get checked out, question everything! Learn your body, know what is best for it and what is not good for it. If you ever have anything close to Stevens-Johnson Syndrome, make sure you go home with the right pain medication. You must at least have the Lidocaine ointment, magic mouthwash, Clobetasol propionate ointment, facial mask, rubber gloves, Dial pump soap, large Band-Aids, Mirasorb Gauze Sponges, and Oxycodone. Have faith and never give up! Hold onto His unchanging hand! He will guide you and protect you! Just know that overnight my life changed—my looks, and everything about me changed. But God spared me and kept me safe! For this, I will never be the same and will forever glorify His Name! I pray this experience will be a blessing and that it will be helpful to someone. Even if this book only helps one person, then I will know I did God's will! God bless you and please, please keep the faith—it may save your life!

May God bless you and enrich your life!

ACKNOWLEDGMENTS

I would like to thank and give honor to my Lord and our Savior Jesus Christ for my life, without whom this would not be possible! Thank you, Lord, for providing me with the vision to take on this project and the drive to complete it. I would like to thank Andre Moore, my husband and best friend, for saving my life and for being with me every day and never leaving my side. Thank you for loving me unconditionally with your whole heart. Thank you to my daughters Renee and Lisa, and my granddaughters Amari and Genesis for your love and care, and for being a lifeline as well! Thank you to Sister Spencer for loving my family and staying with us when I was released from the hospital, for being up in the early mornings with me while I was in pain and encouraging me not to stop, for cooking and cleaning for us, and being there to pray with us! Thank you to my Pastor, Dalyn L. Dunn, and First Lady Dawn Dunn for your support and encouragement. To Deacon and Deaconess Rayford for bringing me home from the hospital and all that you do. To Minister Carmen, Sister Eula, Sister Linda, Sister McIntosh, Sister Nicole, Deacon and Deaconess Terry and Billie, Mia, Tom and Josie, Sister Toni, Sister Zeta, Sister Candice, Sister Deborah, Brother Donyal, and Pastor David Dunn. Thank you to Pastor Dunn's twin Godparents for their prophecies and love. To everyone who brought food or even sent food to our house. Thank you to Sister Royce (Weezy) for the visits and for doing my hair (which took three days since my scalp was burned). Thank you Dalene for taking the pictures and Jaylen for loving and visiting me. Thank you Mom and Ernie for loving me enough and praying for me. Thank you to all my family members from Philadelphia, New Jersey, and Georgia. Thank you family, friends, and Peace Missionary Baptist Church members for not rushing to see me and obeying the doctor's orders, yet sending your love and prayers. Thank you to my Kings Kids for the beautiful cards and words of love you sent me. I will cherish them forever! I love you all to life!

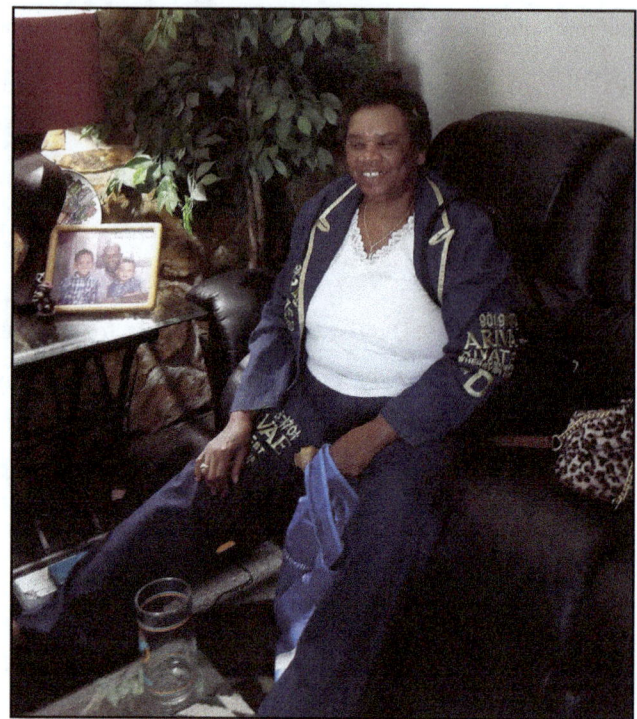

My Mom

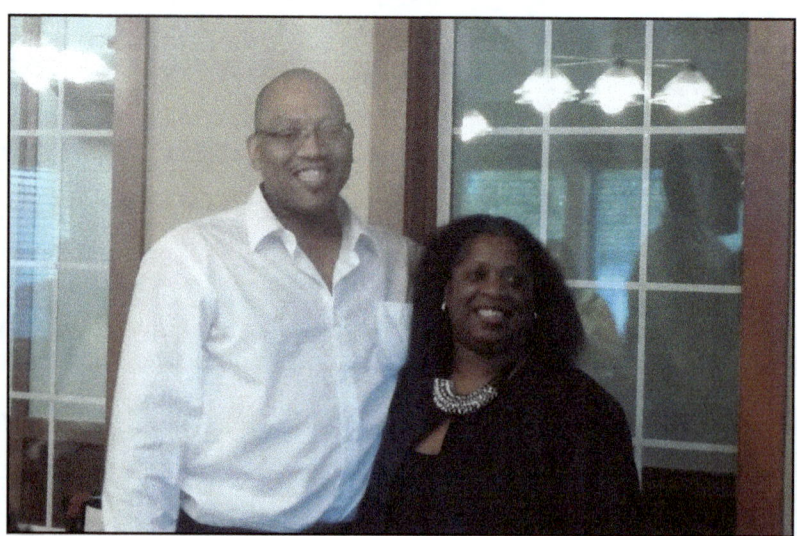

Andre and I when he became an Ordained Deacon

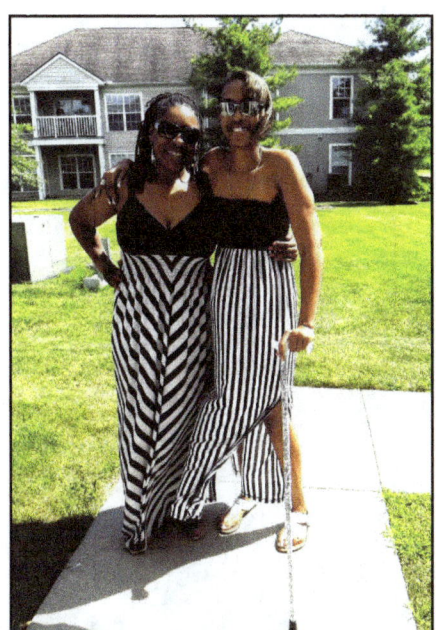
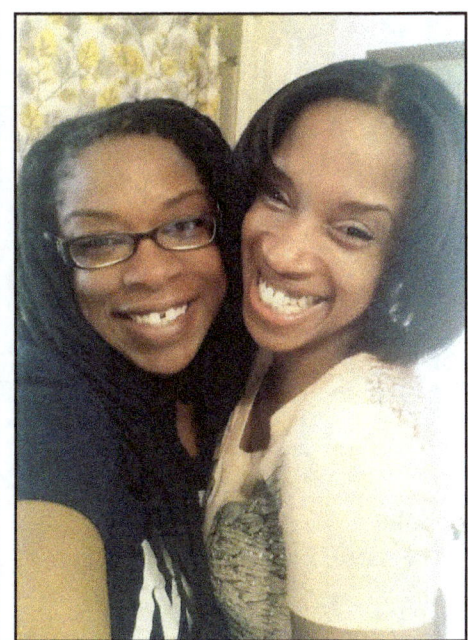

Lisa and Renee

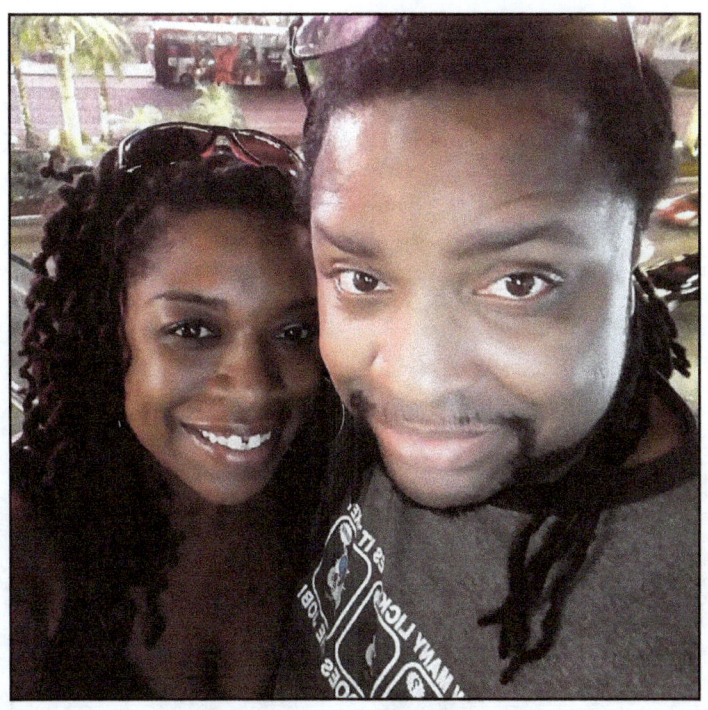

Renee and Marquel

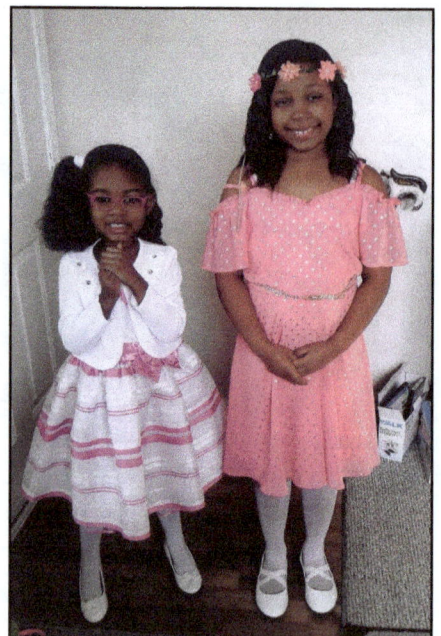
Amari and Genesis

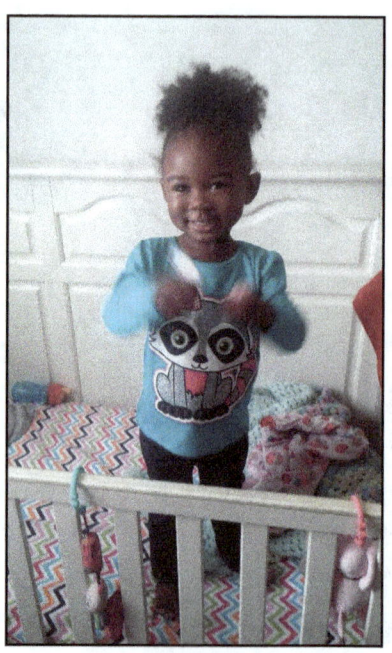
Genesis

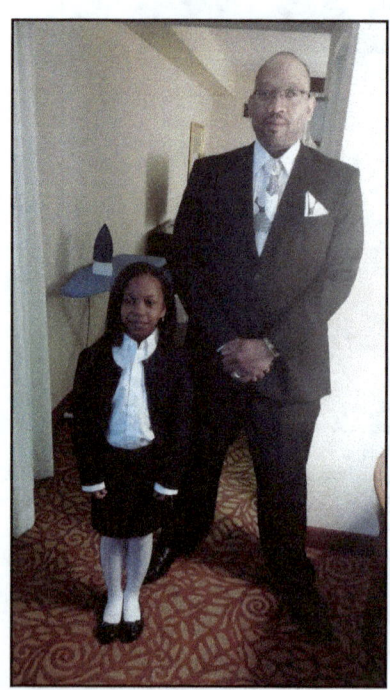
Amari and Andre

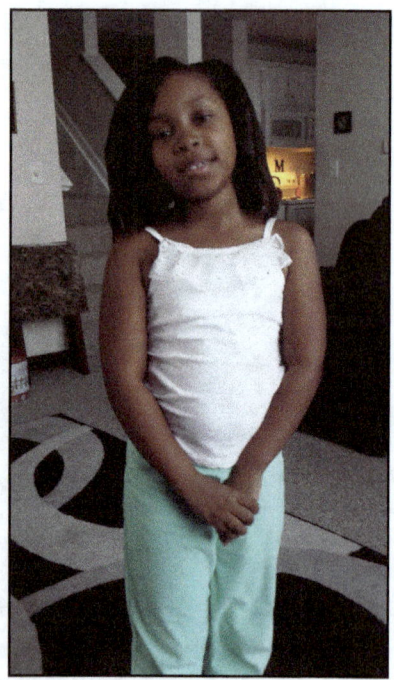
Amari

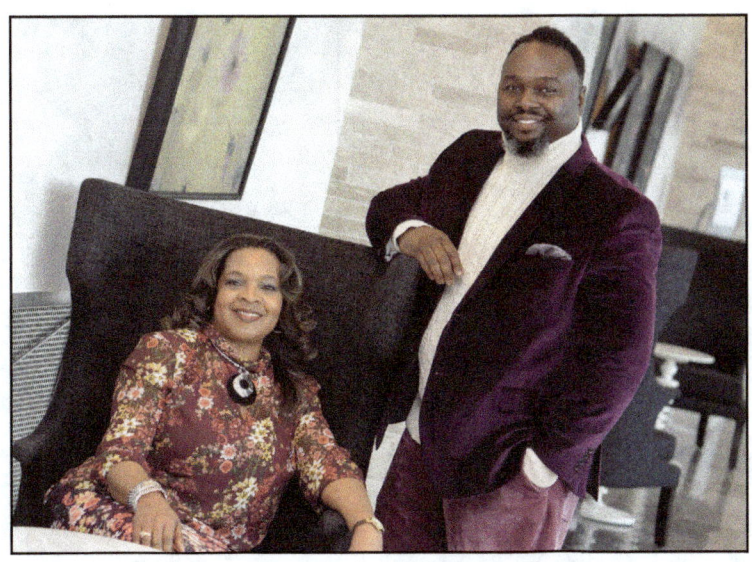

Pastor Dalyn L. Dunn and
First Lady Dawn Dunn

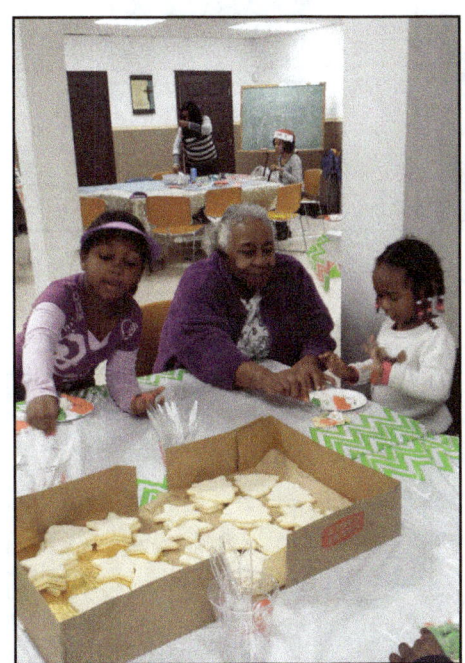

Sister Spencer, Amari and Genesis at the church, with Lisa and Renee in the background

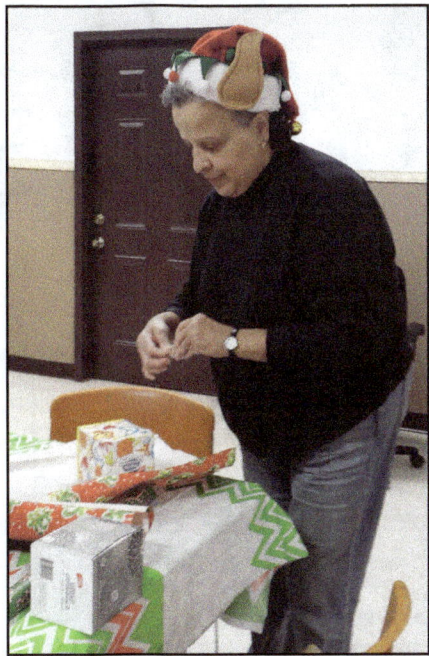

Sister Rayford at the church

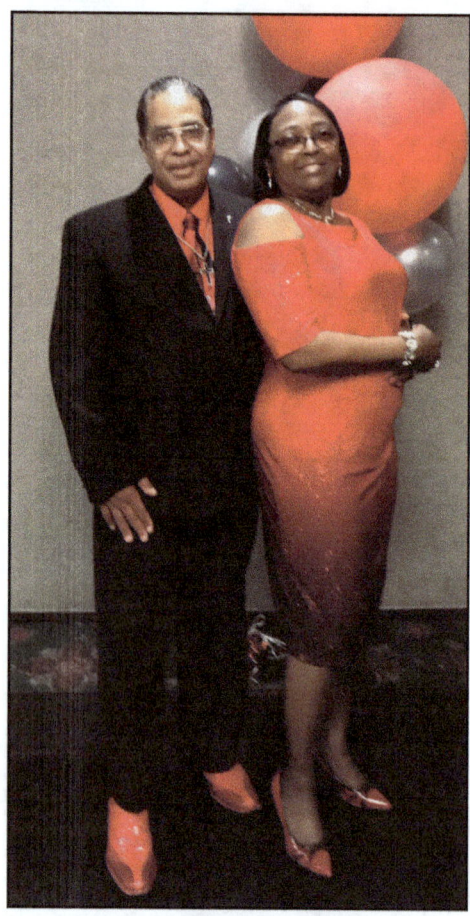

Deacon Terry Graves and
Deaconess Billie Graves

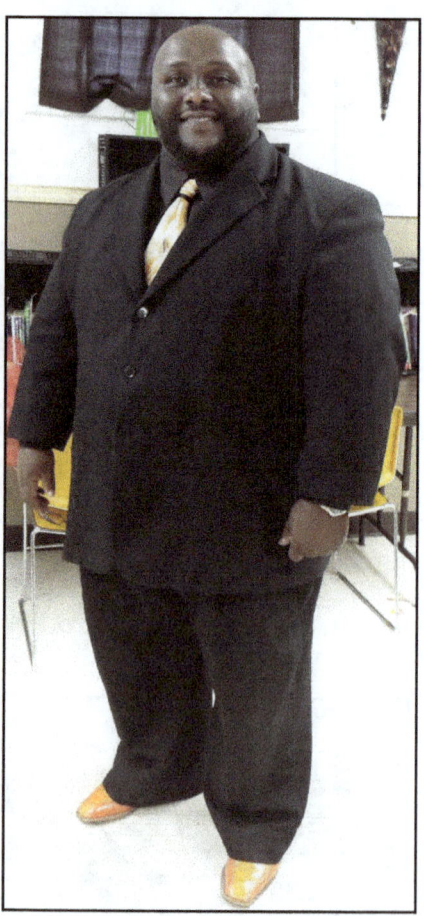

Pastor David Dunn

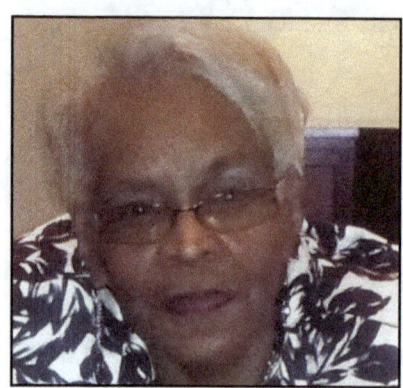

Ms. Eula Stringer

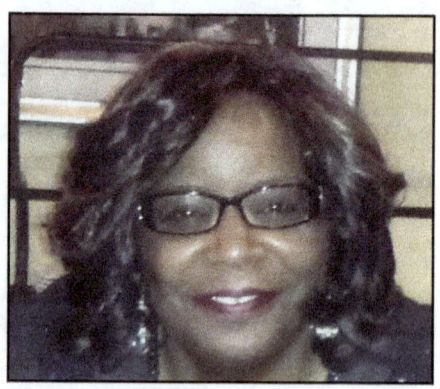

Sister Linda

WHO COULD HAVE IMAGINED!

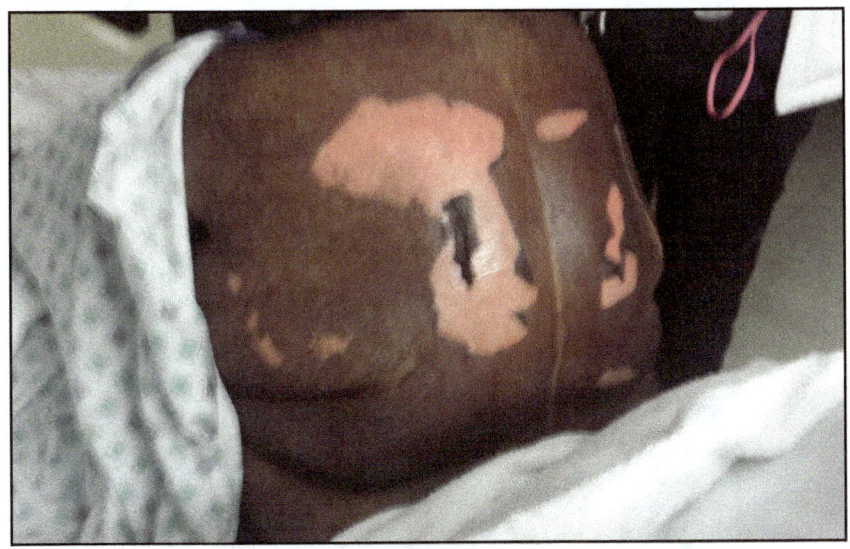

Where Andre touched me and my skin peeled off

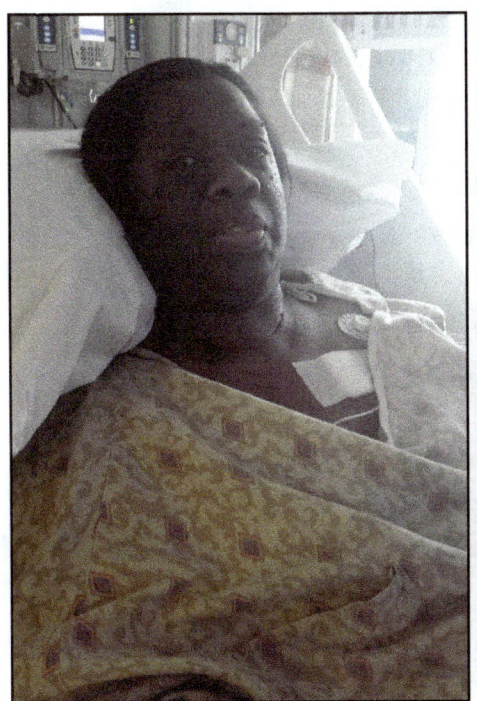

Day two in the hospital before skin blistering started

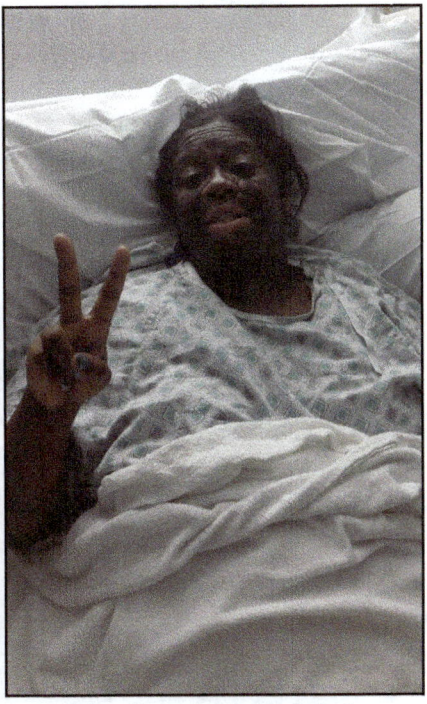

Day three in the hospital

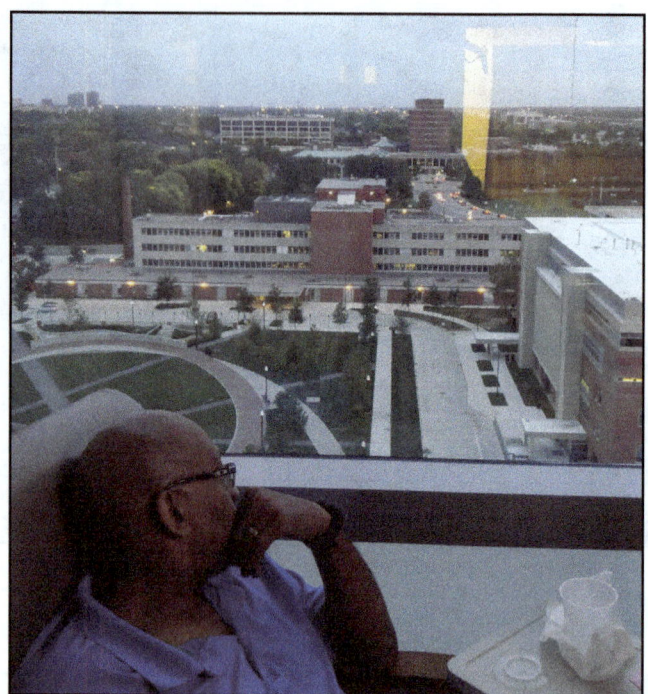
Andre praying and looking out the window

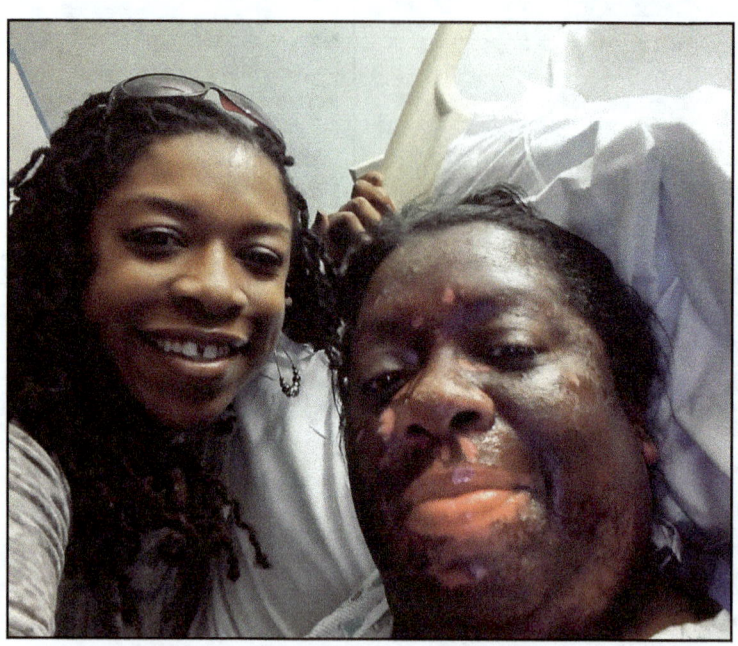
With Renee on day four with swollen face

WHO COULD HAVE IMAGINED!

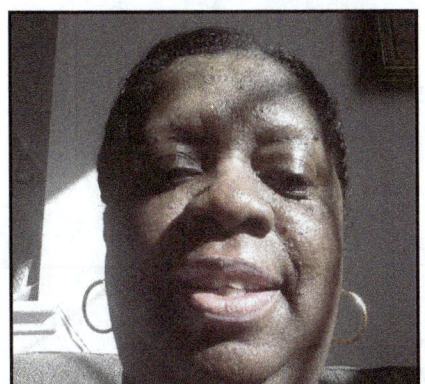
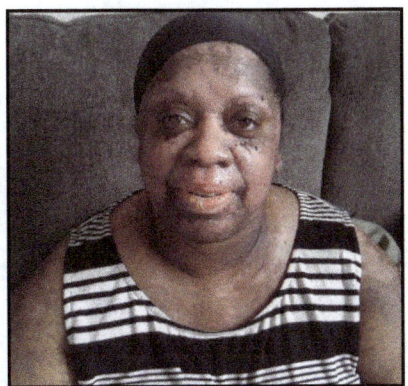

Ready for home

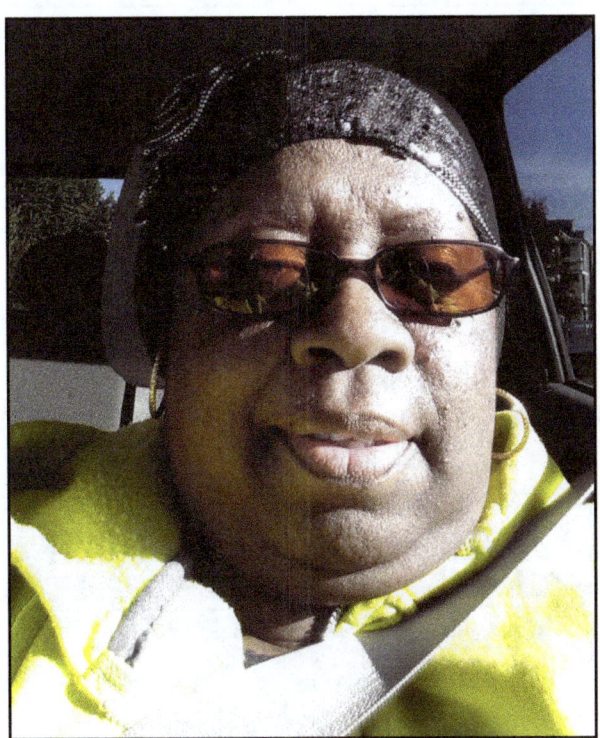

First day outside without mask!

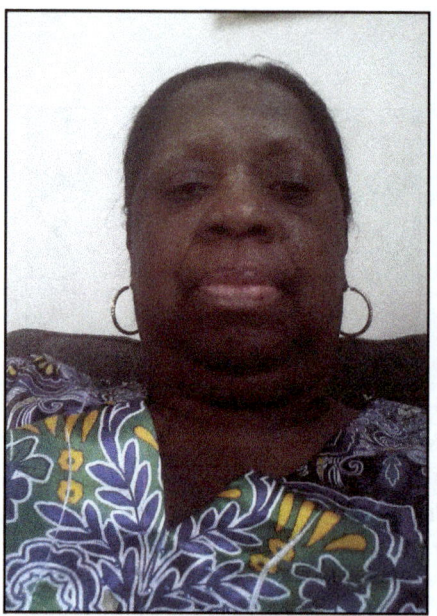
After I got home and started to heal

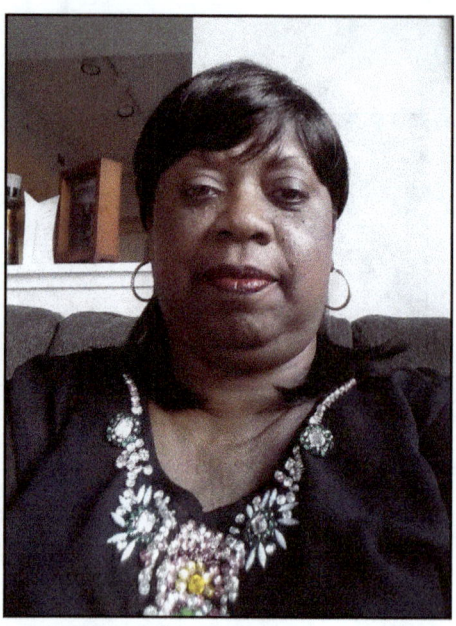
The first day back to church and with my new wig

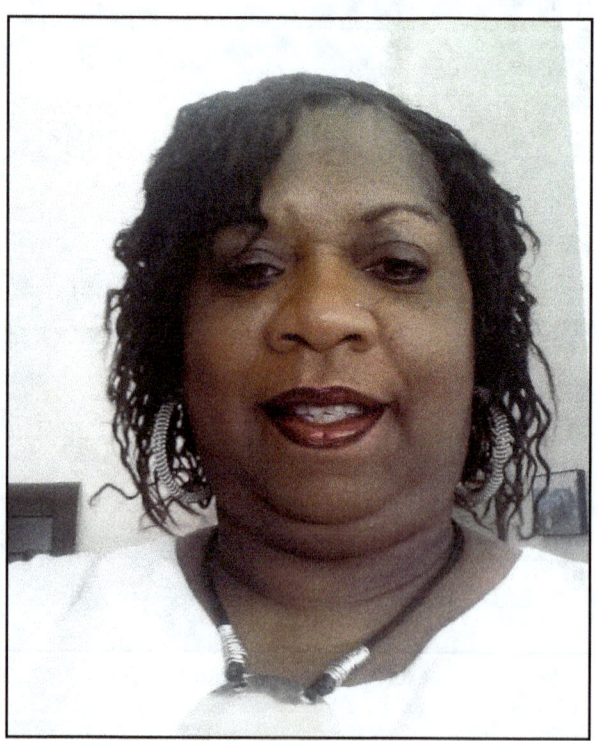
After Royce (Weezy) did my hair

ABOUT THE AUTHOR

Michele Moore was born in Philadelphia, PA as Michele Poland. Throughout her life God has always had His hand on her. She experienced many abnormal situations, but didn't fully recognize them as God's presence. As life went on He continued to uplift, motivate and provide her with hopeful encounters to reveal His presence, purpose and principles. But life was not always positive for Michele, and struggles and trials blocked her view of God's presence and pulled her away from the word of God.

But God had His own agenda; He used her friend Zeta Moore to intercede for her. Zeta introduced Michele to Mt. Herman Baptist Church and Pastor Donald J. Washington. Still, something was missing in her relationship with God. She was not fully focused and did not have the correct attitude to see His presence and the relevance of Him in her life. She was still trying to find her place and desired a deeper relationship with the Father.

A few years later, after leaving Mt. Herman, Michele met up with Pastor Dalyn L. Dunn. He invited her to his church, introduced her to her future husband, and life began to show promise! But she still had that burning desire for a unique relationship with God. Little did she know she was destined to find her purpose and become a blessing by giving back to God!

Be careful what you ask of God, because He might give you exactly what you desire.

Michele never could have imagined that the close relationship with God she'd prayed so hard for would come through Stevens-Johnson Syndrome. She shares her pain and suffering in this book as part of her journey through this illness with God, and hopes that her experiences and those of her family inspire readers to listen when God speaks.

Today Michele lives in Columbus, Ohio and attends Peace Missionary Baptist Church where the honorable Dalyn L. Dunn, MACM is the pastor. She is a Deaconess and is married to Deacon Andre Moore. She and their family, daughters Lisa and Renee, and granddaughters Amari and Genesis, love and cherish their relationship with God as well as the entire Peace family.

Michele now knows how to trust God, go where He sends her, do what He says to do, say what He says to say, give when and where He says to give, and listen when He says, "Be still and be quiet!"

Please keep our Peace family in your prayers so that some of the proceeds of this book will future our work in the Kingdom of God!

www.ingramcontent.com/pod-product-compliance
Lightning Source LLC
LaVergne TN
LVHW021600070426
835507LV00014B/1881